Blind but Not Broken:
A Story of a Sinner Saved by God's Grace

by

Briston Bradley

Blind But Not Broken Copyright 2018 by Briston Bradley

ISBN: 9781793320315

All rights reserved. No part of this publication may be reproduced, stored in a retrieval system or transmitted, in any form, or by any means, electronic, mechanical, recorded, photocopied, or otherwise, without the prior written permission of both the copyright owner and the above-mentioned publisher of this book, except by a reviewer who may quote brief passages in a review.

The scanning, uploading, and distribution of this book via the Internet or via any other means without the permission of the publisher is illegal and punishable by law. Please purchase only authorized electronic editions and do not participate in or encourage electronic piracy of copy written materials.

First Edition: December 2018

Lenox Avenue Publishing

www. lenoxavenuepublishing.virb.com

Printed in the United States of America

Thank You and Dedication to:

Kingdom Builders Outreach C.O.G.I.C.

Mom and Grandparents

My Family

Let Go and Let God Anointed Ministries

Special Thanks and Dedication to:

Greater Works Christian Church

My children - Joe Stewart, Trevin Bradley, Londyn Maye, Iris Bradley

and my Wife and Love Phoebe Bradley

Table of Contents

Chapter 1: My Beginnings 5
Chapter 2: Young Adulthood 17
Chapter 3: Spiritual Gifts 29
Chapter 4: The Accident 37
Chapter 5: Hospital Stay 49
Chapter 6: Accepting My New Life as a Blind Man ... 53
Chapter 7: Answering the Call 59
Chapter 8: The Future Looks Brighter Than Ever ... 65

Chapter 1: My Beginnings
Jeremiah 1:5

I was born during a time when a lot was going on in black communities throughout the country. Like other black boys and girls born during that time, I am a post-Civil Rights era child who did not have to suffer through much of what my grandparents or even my parents had to endure. Yet and still, the hardship of being a black boy did not escape me. My mom gave birth to me in 1989 in Benton, Arkansas and although she was my mother it would be many years before I could truly embrace her as that in my life. My grandmother raised me and, in my eyes, she was my momma. My parents where teenagers when I was born. My father had just graduated from high school and my mother was a senior by the time I came along.

Although the shame of being a single teen mother wasn't as bad in 1989 as it had been decades before, my grandmother still wanted to make sure I had some stability in my life while she encouraged her daughter (my mother) to pursue higher education after high school. So, off to college my mother went leaving me behind with my grandparents as an infant. My dad didn't even have a second thought about pursuing his dreams and off to the Army Reserves he went. I was now officially an American statistic – a black boy born to a single mother and being raised by his grandparents. That was my introduction to life.

I recall having visits from my mother here and there but couldn't really comprehend why she'd left me behind. It bothered me as a kid. I didn't care that she went into the Army National Guard and was busy serving the country. She should have been home serving me was all I thought. That was the seed of pent up anger and bitterness towards her that began to grow inside of me. Although my parents weren't really in the picture, my grandmother and grandfather did the best they could to raise me. I am eternally grateful for their love, support and strength. They lived in a country town in Arkansas called Prattsville and there wasn't much to do there. But us kids who lived in Prattsville made a way to have fun anyway. Our home was so deep into the country that if I'd walk through a field that was near the house, I'd easily come upon a pond for fishing and plenty of woods for hunting.

The first time I went hunting with my grandfather was when I was just five years old. Even at that young age, I felt a sense of power charge through my small body when I held that heavy rifle. Knowing that I could take down an animal with the pull of the trigger from my little hands was surreal. Hunting and fishing were relaxing for me even at that young age. Although I no longer hunt, fishing still gives me a chance to be at peace with my own thoughts and imagination. There is something about the energy of water that does your spirit and mind well. My grandfather taught me the responsibilities of hunting and I fell in love with it at an early age. I didn't have my first deer kill until I was around eleven or twelve, but the years leading up to it that I spent with my grandfather in those woods were priceless.

Like so many black boys growing up without a father, my introduction into manhood came through my grandfather. Not only did he teach me how to shoot a rifle at five but also how to start and work a lawnmower at that age as well. I was so little, that I'd have to start the rider mower first and then jump in the seat to steer it across the lawn. Granddaddy taught me how to chop wood for our wood burning stove, sand cars, and put up fences around the property for our horses that were in the pasture. I was raised as a country boy who knew how to do some things with his hands. I still think every young man should know how to do something with their hands other than harming another or getting into trouble.

As a kid that was living in the country, I would find things to do that would keep me busy and entertained. There were no shopping malls or movie theaters close by to go to so you had to make the best of what was available. For example, I had a love for music from very young and taught myself how to play the drums. I didn't own a drum set but would grab a couple of my grandmother's wooden spoons and would beat them up against some of the empty five-gallon buckets we had around the house. My grandmother would cook big meals on the weekends and play church music throughout the house while she was doing it. That was my cue to play my makeshift drums to the music playing. My grandmother would get so mad at me because hearing my bucket banging was messing up her worship time. I didn't care though because the timing and rhythm of my playing that came natural for me had gotten better the more I did it. Her gospel music was a perfect accompaniment to my drumming.

Like any black kid living in the country with their grandparents, I had to go to church every Sunday. My grandfather may have been the man of the house but Jesus Christ was the King of it. I enjoyed the services and although I was only about seven, I felt that I needed to give my life to God. One Sunday morning, while the preacher gave the altar call, I marched right up front and told him that I wanted to be baptized. My grandparents were happy and praising God for my decision. I knew that I was different than most kids my age and felt a calling on my life although I couldn't comprehend all that it meant. So, giving my life to Christ was for me a way of acknowledging that call.

Although I was a young kid, I knew that I loved God and wanted to serve Him. I remember the ride home after the service where I gave my life to him to be one filled with joy. As we walked into our four-bedroom country house the strangest thing happened though. As I walked past the washing machine it all of a sudden began to shake. My grandparents had walked past the machine before me and nothing happened, but it started moving as I approached it. Keep in mind, the machine was not turned on which made it even more strange. When it began to shake, my grandmother looked at my grandfather and said to him, "Ain't nobody mad but the devil". That was my first introduction to the supernatural realm, but it would not be the last. Two weeks after that incident things got even stranger for me.

My grandparents had a modest home, but because there were four bedrooms, I was able to have my own room. It was down the hall from theirs and they slept with the door closed and so did I. They were in their mid-forties and needed their privacy which was understandable. One evening, I decided to sleep with the bible under my pillow which is something I had done from time to time. Now remember, I was only seven years old but knew that God's word was sacred and wanted it as close to me as possible as I slept. I remember waking up around 12:29 a.m. and for the next minute I heard time change as the clock hit 12:30 a.m. It is hard to explain, but I heard time shift. Right after that my bed began to vibrate and then it raised about six inches off of the ground. All of a sudden, the closet doors got knocked off the hinges and the mirror on the right side of my bed fell off the wall and shattered on the floor. The bed then hit the ground and my bedroom door flew open. I jumped out of bed and literally flew down to my grandparent's bedroom.

I remember being upset and yelling, "Grandmother, it's after me, don't let it get me!". Grandma got up with the anointing oil and went into my bedroom to rebuke whatever spirit that was in my room. All I heard was her flinging the oil in the room and telling whatever it was to get out and that it couldn't have me. From that day forward my grandmother would always remind others that I was called from birth and was different than others. After that incident, I asked my grandparents to move me to one of the other bedrooms which they did. Although they'd still sleep with their doors closed, I would get up to open it in the middle of the night to make me feel safer. Thankfully, another incident like that one never happened again.

I still enjoyed going to church with my grandparents during my younger years but that began to change a bit when I entered my high school years. I was always a pretty active guy and was a natural at sports. I was on the basketball team as a point guard and the football team as a receiver, tailback and kickoff returner. I was fast too and ran a 4.4-second forty-yard sprint. You would have thought that some college would have recruited me just on speed alone but that didn't happen. By this time my father was a bit more involved in my life and lived in Pine Bluff,

Arkansas. Pine Bluff had more going on than Prattsville and I liked going up there to hang out on weekends. I didn't make it there every weekend, but when I did, I partied, drank and smoked weed. By the time I hit my senior year in high school, I was a pro at guzzling down gin followed by smoking some blunts. Partying now replaced my love for the church.

My circle of friends in Pine Bluff were to say the least some pretty shady characters, but I didn't care. We wanted money, girls and fun in abundance. I had access to all of that when I decided to join the Folks Nation gang which is affiliated with the Crips. Folk Nation was started in 1978 in Chicago and quickly spread throughout the mid-west and south within a decade. The gang was formidable in Arkansas during my high school years and I was a proud member. I was into drugs, violence and just about anything else the gang wanted me to get involved in. During the week I was my grandmother's sweet boy who was still living with her, but on the weekends when I wasn't with her, I was a hell raiser. To make it even crazier, my father was a police officer who had no idea of the double life I was living. I was smart enough not to have any gang emblems tattooed on my body, just my street name. Being a police officer, I knew that if he'd saw anything on my body or around me that was gang-related he'd give me hell.

Making sure I kept my grades up was important to me because I didn't want to give my grandmother any reason to worry as to whether or not I'd graduate from high school. I managed to get accepted into the University of Arkansas, major in Kinesiology and join the National Guard. Although I liked college, it just wasn't for me and I quit in order to work and make some money because I was also a new father who needed to support his daughter. I loved making money and life was going well for me at this point. One day I had stopped by my father's house to speak with a relative that was staying there off and on. My father wasn't home because he was overseas working a job. By the time I got back to work I realized that I had left my cell phone at his house so I called another relative who lived not far from my dad's place and asked if they could bring it to me. She agreed and headed over to his house. Just as she pulled up, a man walked up to her and asked her to sign for a package that was to be delivered to my father's home. My relative didn't think anything of it, signed for it and left it in the house. Things got really crazy after that for her though.

Unbeknownst to her, the house was under police surveillance for several weeks. Now keep in mind, my dad had no idea about this because he was out of the country. As soon as my relative left the house to head over to my job with my phone, she was followed by local and state police and got pulled over. Shocked and confused with sirens blasting and lights flashing, she had no idea what was going on. The police informed her that the package she signed for contained drugs and cash. As a matter of fact, it was exactly twenty-two pounds of marijuana and $18,000 in cash. She had let them know that she was on her way to give me my phone and they immediately thought the package was for me. They told her that they wanted to speak with me and find out if I was involved in this or not.

As soon as the relative got to my job I could see that she was very angry. Not knowing if I had anything to do with it, she told me that the police wanted to talk to me. I assured her that I was innocent and not involved at all in having drugs delivered to my dad's house. I mean, what kind of fool would I be to even do anything like that wide in the open? Besides, my dad was former law enforcement and when it came to stuff like that he did not play. If it was my stuff, I would have had it delivered to another address before I'd even tried something like that with him. Although I had been involved in gang activities and selling of weed here and there, I had no idea about that package. I assured the relative that everything would be fine because I was innocent.

The next day, the cops showed up on my job and began interrogating me like a convicted criminal. They'd let me know that they had been watching the house for some time and that my phone was tapped. They obviously had nothing on me because they spent more time trying to intimidate me in order to put fear in me. They wanted to get me to confess to something. It didn't work. While they were playing their bad cop act, an older black couple that had been watching the whole episode asked if I was ok and told the police their actions were not warranted. Till this day, I'm grateful for that couple although I never got their names. I was only nineteen years old, but the police didn't care. They asked for my car keys and then proceeded to ransack through my care like rapid dogs looking for a steak. They were so ignorant and never apologized for throwing my belongings on the ground. After finding nothing, they let me alone and went their way.

I didn't like the police and didn't like being treated like a criminal by them. It turns out that whoever sent that package was using my dad's address as a drop off point because for the most part no one was ever home. It was easy for the drug dealers to use that address and not have the package belongings traced back to them. Not even two years later, the two dudes involved in that scheme were shot and killed. That whole incident had me shook a bit. It was the beginning of some serious life decisions I was about to make in the next few years.

Chapter 2: Young Adulthood
Matthew 6:24

Like I said before, ever since I was a little boy, I knew that I had a call upon my life, a call to serve in the ministry. My grandparents, mother and a host of other relatives knew it and liked to remind me of it. Although I was involved with the gang, I still loved God and serving Him in any way I could when I did go to church and even outside of the church. Whether it was helping someone out less fortunate than me or singing in the church choir, any service to God was rewarding. My grandmother raised me to always put my trust in the Lord and do right no matter what circumstances I may find myself in. I was raised with a good set of morals and conscience. I had good examples around me as well. My mother and father were both former military soldiers with my dad building a career as a police officer. You would have thought with that great of a moral foundation I would stay on the straight and narrow and follow a righteous path from early on, but it didn't.

I enjoyed having nice things and I knew that nice things required money. Some of the people I'd be hanging around wore the latest styles, drove the newest cars and kept a roll of cash in their pocket. I wanted that life. College wasn't going to get it to me fast enough so I took the quick route, I got into the drug game. Now, I was no drug kingpin like Carlos Escobar dealing in cocaine. My way of making some easy money was by selling weed. Many of my friends were doing it and although I had a mind of my own, I wanted in on the game. It's funny to see now that corporations are raising millions of dollars to get in on the cannabis industry, but when we were doing it, we'd be locked up for carrying as little bit of an amount as a joint. Times are truly changing.

I had a steady flow of customers and what most people would make in two weeks on a fulltime job, I'd make it in just three hours. It was fast money. A lot of the dudes I knew who sold made sure they stayed styled up in urban gear like Coogi or Phat Farm, but not me. I was a polished dope boy who preferred wearing designer clothes like Ralph Lauren, Tommy Hilfiger and what I'd like to call "pretty boy" clothes.

I was country on the inside but a stylish street brother on the outside. It made me stand out from the others and brought some haters my way. I was cautious about how I handled business because of it. Never would I let any customers come to my home to buy, I'd make sure if they said they were referred to me I'd check with the one who referred me to make sure it wasn't a set up. My dad was a cop and I knew how they'd move so I wasn't about to be caught. I still held a job at a grocery store when I started out but soon quit because I was making much more money in the street. I was a pretty good dice player too and would win no less than $2500 anytime I'd play. I enjoyed the money that came with the streets but I didn't like the negativity that you had to deal with along with it.

My family had no idea about the double life I was living. I remember a few times I'd be drunk and high in church while singing in the choir. I knew how to cover up my inebriation pretty well in order to fool the most discerning in church. In my mind, I wasn't being disrespectful to God or the church, I was just being me. I thought it would be more of a hypocrite of me to be all up in church like I was a saint and pretended like I never did anything wrong. To me that's being a hypocrite, a fake. So, if I felt like hitting a blunt before service or taking a shot of gin, I'd do it. It helped me to relax and actually, in my mind, connect with spiritually a bit better while in service.

Little by little my life was starting to spiral out of control. I had money in my pocket and fancy designer clothes, but there was no peace. Life for me was more about hustling and looking over my shoulders. I carried a gun with me for protection and had to pull it out a few times to ward off other dudes who would try to test my courage. I remember one time I had attended this fraternity party and had my gun on me like I always do. There were some guys there that knew I always had money and weed on me. As I left the party to go and get into my car, I hadn't noticed that these same dudes were parked three cars behind me, waiting for me to come outside. I recognized them while I was in the party because of some past issues we'd had with each other. I finally noticed them as they stepped out of their car and knew they were up to no good. As soon as I knew what was up, I pulled my gun and pointed it at them. They pulled their guns and pointed it at me, paused and took cover. That brief pause and them scrambling for cover gave me the few seconds I needed to get in my car and take off. They chased me for a while but I eventually was able to out maneuver them and get away.

I had set out to have a good time that evening and mind my business. It ended up with my life being threatened.

That night showed me that more than ever, being in the street game had a whole bunch of problems. That night also showed me how real things could get but it wasn't the last time death came knocking. I had been living in my father's trailer home but unfortunately, a fire destroyed it which meant I had to move into a hotel until I could find my own spot.

One night, I went to a nearby McDonald's and pulled into the drive thru to place my order. I was in my truck and had a friend with me in the passenger's seat. All of a sudden, as I was placing my order through the order box, a car pulled up beside mine, then another car behind that one. I usually kept my gun with me but didn't have it that night because I'd figure since the McDonald's was behind the hotel there was no need to carry it because we wouldn't be out for long. I looked at the occupants in the car and stared them down, they did the same to me. I calmly ordered my food, paid for it and headed back to the hotel. They began to follow me. Just as I pulled into the hotel parking lot I jumped out and was ready to confront and fight them.

That's when my passenger yelled "They got a gun!". I jumped back into the car and took off. They chased me and tried to drive me off the road but I was able to escape. I am not sure if they really had a gun or not but if they did, I know if I had my pistol on me gun fire would have been exchanged.

There have been times when I could sense I was being set up for a robbery or killing. Thank God my instincts were correct and I got out of those places before they could do what they set out to do. Even though I was doing my own thing and being wild in the streets, God was still protecting me. Once, a dude put a gun to my head and pulled the trigger but the gun jammed and the bullet didn't fire. Several times I had dudes to jump me and start fighting.

I remember one time when I had been jumped, the guys who did it got away with $3000 they took from me. That really pissed me off because now they were messing up my income. The thug in me wouldn't let them get away with it either. Later on, I dressed in all black and went to the house I knew they'd be at. My car was black so in a sense I was in stealth mode in order to retaliate. I had some buddies with me who had known they jacked me for my money. We were ready to fight. I found the house, walked up to the front door and knocked. I grabbed the guy who opened the door and threw him outside with me and beat him to a pulp. We then went inside and got the money they had stolen. I wasn't a type of guy to start any trouble, but when you came and started it with me best believe I wasn't about to let you get away with it.

My life was quickly spiraling out of control. Deep down inside I knew I needed to stop doing what I was doing and lead a life without all of the drama. That was easier said than done though. When you are making large sums of money, have people fear you and can gain access to whatever you want the ego takes over. My ego led me down some dark and dangerous roads but I was too headstrong to just turn everything around. I knew that the end of the type of life I was living was either prison or the graveyard, but the money was too good to stop it on a dime. At times I cared and promised myself that I was going to end this troubled lifestyle. I didn't want to be known as dope boy for the rest of my life. I also wanted to be around to raise my daughter and leave a positive impression on her. Having a child in your life that you love and care about can give you a wakeup call like no other. Well, at least it would do that for the average person. The thing about men and women who are involved in illegal activities is this, they are primarily concerned about themselves and anyone else comes second, third or last.

My wakeup call came when an uncle in another city called to tell me that I needed to slow my life down because he had heard about me in the streets. I was building a reputation as a tough guy who was primarily focused on making a lot of money. Not too long after he gave me a warning, his warning came to past. One day I was at a stop light and a car pulled up beside me. I knew the driver was an enemy and always kept a gun on him. My mind was ready to battle it out with him but I had my baby daughter in the car with me. I know if this dude pulled out his gun and started shooting, I'd pull mine out and start shooting which means my daughter would have possibly been caught on in the crossfire and shot. I kept my cool and just looked straight ahead at the light and at him out of the side view of my eye. Fortunately for me and my daughter, he never turned his head to catch a glimpse of me and moved on when the light turned green. I was thanking God that at that moment, my life and the life of my child were spared! That is something I will never forget.

That incident turned out to be the best thing to happen to me. It was the beginning of me trying to turn my life around but first I had to renounce my gang affiliation. Anyone who knows anything about gangs knows that once you get in, it is nearly impossible to get out. When I had informed my leaders that I wanted out they initially said they understood and gave me the ok to walk away. But unfortunately, they had a change a heart. They reminded me that the only way out was death, and even prison doesn't even exempt you from your gang affiliation. I knew that I wasn't afraid of death because I had so many close calls to it which let them know that I had a higher purpose than running the streets. I had let them know that if they wanted to kill me, so be it but I was out. I left on bad terms with them and didn't care because I knew if they didn't kill me, the streets eventually would do it if I did not turn my life around.

It was a miracle that I was able to hide my street life away from my family. I've always been a pretty charismatic guy and good talker so even if they did confront me about it, I knew how to talk my way out of it. My family knew that I was a gambler, but that's about it. I believe that around this time in my life God started to work on my heart and give me a disdain for the streets. The things that use to appeal to me where starting to lose its glitter. I still loved having money in my pocket, but the problems that came with it was nothing short of evil. I didn't have peace, had to always look over my shoulder and ran from death every day. That's no way for a young man to live.

People often glamorize the gangster life. You see it in movies and young boys want to grow up to immolate characters like *Scarface* or the gangsters in *The Godfather*. What these young boys and men don't understand is that often, these tough gangsters end up gunned down or serving the rest of their lives in prison. They don't see the paranoia and depression that wreaks hell upon your mind and emotions. They don't see how lonely that life really can be. I had friends, but I also know that with the right price any one of them could turn on me in a heartbeat. One mistake could cost me my life including trusting the wrong person. The wrong person could turn me into the police or set me up for danger. You live your life as if you're a fugitive, ready to leave town at any given moment if the pressure was too much. That's not a way to live, it's not the life God intended for anybody to live.

There is a dark side to being a gang-banger, drug dealer and street hustler. None of them will lead you to a life worth bragging about at the end of your life. I didn't want my memory with my daughter and future children to be that their father was a street thug who died too young. I want to leave a legacy for my children and that required to begin to walk a righteous path. Too many black children are raised without their fathers in their lives. I did not want my children to be a part of that statistic. I know what it was like not to have parents daily interacting in your life. My parents were good people and hard workers, but neither of them raised me. Perhaps if they had been around to co-parent me, I may have not chosen the streets, but maybe not. Looking back on it now I believe that I had to go through that gangster life and get it out of my system.

I believe my daughter was my inspiration to change my life around. Now don't get me wrong, it didn't happen overnight like you see in the movies. There was a lot of going back and forth between me and God. I knew that my best option was to find my way back to the Lord. Just because I was in the street life didn't mean that the God life left me. That's the thing about a calling, it never leaves you. In the book of Romans in the Bible it says, *"For the gifts and calling of God are without repentance"*. What that means is that when God has given you a divine gift or has a call on your life to serve Him, it is not revoked. You can run from it all you want, but it will eventually come to pass. God will use whatever He needs to get your attention. For me, it was the possibility of my daughter being shot up in my car because of my foolishness. An innocent baby shouldn't have to pay for my decisions and mistakes. My divine call was still on my life with every bag of weed I sold, every shot of gin I drank and every person I beat up with my fists. God didn't see me any different than if I was in a pulpit preaching for Him. I was His no matter what I did, He wasn't going to let me go. I had a destiny to fulfill and whether I liked it or not, it was going to be happen.

If you are reading this book and are caught up in that thug life, I encourage you to pause and think about is it all worth it. How do you want your children to remember you? At the end of the day, you have one life to live and one legacy to give. Make the choice to do right because all that other stuff will lead you to darkness and hopelessness.

Chapter 3: Spiritual Gifts
Ephesians 4:11

Life has a way of bringing you into your purpose without you realizing it. I believe that everything happens for a reason, whether it's for the good or bad. There are hardly any coincidences. It especially works this way when you have a call of God upon your life. You may think you have plans to go in one direction for your life, but low and behold, God shows up to put you right on the path you clearly need to be on.

I knew that my life was set apart for something special to do and no matter what was going on around me, I saw the hand of God at work. I remember one time I was riding in the car with a cousin. I had a good amount of weed on me that I was going to sell and we had been smoking some as well. I believe it was around the fourth of July and we were heading out to an event. You know during the holidays the police have check points set up to capture any drunk drivers, people with outstanding warrants or traffic violations, and any drug users or dealers like me riding around with drugs. I knew in my spirit that I had to get the weed out of my car and secure it in a safe place before we headed over to the event. My cousin didn't sense what I was sensing. Something in my spirit was telling me to get my car cleaned out of any drugs. But my cousin kept badgering me about not being paranoid and to just head over to the event. For a moment I listened to him and was heading over to the event but my spirit kept letting me know that it would have been a big mistake to do so without first getting the drugs out of my car.

After going back and forth with him, I decided to follow my instincts and drop the marijuana off first, make sure there was no smell of weed in the car and then head over to the event. It pissed my cousin off just for a moment because he thought we were wasting precious time we could have spent partying. After I cleaned out the car, we headed out and we approached one of those police road blocks. Wouldn't you know it my car was stopped and thoroughly checked! If I had not listened to what my spirit was telling me, we would have ended up in jail. After they searched the car and found nothing, we were allowed to go. My cousin was blown away at how I knew to instinctively use precaution. I'd let him know that my spirit does not lead me wrong and trust me whenever I said something doesn't feel right. I avoided a lot of problems and headaches that day. Even today, if something doesn't feel right to me, I am not going to do it. I thank God for that gift of discernment.

There was another incident when I was coming back from a military funeral with some of my fellow buddies from the reserves. I was the only one in a suit, the others had on their military attire, but not dress uniforms. I was hesitant to get in the car with these guys, something was discouraging me from doing so. Rather than obey that prompting, I jumped into the car anyway. There were four of us and I was sitting behind the driver. Two of the passengers had weed on them because we had been smoking in the car. Out of nowhere, there was a state trooper trailing our car with his police lights on signaling for us to pull over. He approached the car, and boy were we nervous. The guys with the weed on them had to eat it and one of them hid a half smoked joint in his sock. It was too late to get the smell of marijuana out of the car and the cop who approached us said he'd smelled it as he leaned into the car.

We told him we were coming back from a fellow soldier's funeral and even showed him the obituary from the service. That did not move him. All of a sudden, he looked in the back seat right into my face, but said nothing. I calmly looked back at him, not trying to lose eye contact which would make him think I was guilty of something. After he ran the plates and driver's license, he said he was letting us go with a warning for speeding and that the only reason why he believed we were at a funeral was because I was wearing a dark suit. That officer didn't realize that what he saw was not a man in a suit, but a man with a call on his life and out of the goodness of his heart he'd let us go. Once again, I avoided being arrested because I'm sure he would have if he found that half joint tucked in the sock of one of the passengers. When it comes to black males, they will arrest the whole group and then sort it out later.

There have been so many times I know the hand of God protected me from danger. I remember once I was hanging out with a fellow church drummer. We were headed to a church event out of town. Although we were musicians in the church, we were still doing our dirt in the streets which is why we probably bonded. I had left my car back home and was riding with him when he decided to stop and see some friends of his. The house was full of shady characters not to mention that there were drugs, guns and money out open on the table. I already knew what they were about but kept my cool. We had only been there for a short time when my friend got a call from some woman. He let me know that he was going to head over to see her and for me to just sit tight. Keep in mind, I didn't know these people and by the looks of things they were ready to set things off if they thought I may have been up to no good. With my friend now gone off to go see this woman, I was left to keep my cool and composure around these dudes.

After about two hours of waiting I called my friend to see when he was planning to come back to pick me up. Would you believe that he said he wasn't coming back and was spending the night with the woman because she didn't want him to go! I was hotter than fish grease! I didn't know these dudes in this house and didn't have a weapon on me in case something started to pop off. Needless to say, I did not sleep a wink that night and stayed awake while sitting up in a chair. That night showed me that I had to change my life. Even being half way committed to church wasn't going to be enough. I had to be committed all the way. It was around this time that the reality of my circumstances really started to come into focus. I was making money selling drugs but had no financial security. Here I was a father with nothing to leave behind to my daughter if something were to happen to me. My transition out of the street life began, or at least it began in my mind.

It was around this time that I had decided to pay my grandparents a visit. I was still close to them but now that I was an adult, I had my own life and didn't see them as often as I'm sure they would have liked. I will never forget the day. It was a Friday and upon arriving at their home I saw a whole bunch of my relatives in the yard enjoying a barbeque. I had no idea they had a cookout going on and it was a pleasant surprise. I saw cousins, and other relatives. I was as happy to see them as they were as happy to see me. It was a sight to behold. While I was there, I spent some time talking with my grandmother at her kitchen table. She expressed concern about my fast lifestyle and wanted me to commit fully to Jesus Christ. She said that she was going to keep praying for me and that she had did her best to steer me and some of my cousins into the right direction.

My grandmother seemed hurt that I had not adhere to her directions and went into a whole other direction for my life. Her words pierced my heart and I began to cry. It was not a sad cry but one of surrender. Just one tear fell from my face but it was full of years of regret. I did not want my grandmother to be disappointed with me. She was not just my grandmother but my mother. She was the woman who had raised me to know right from wrong. I was her heart but my actions were breaking it.

The next day, Saturday, I was reflecting on seeing my family and the talk I had with my grandmother. I knew she was right and that God used her to remind me that I had a greater call on my life. The road I was heading down was dark and lonely. There was to be no good outcome if I kept doing the mess I was doing. This had to stop. I had decided that the next day, Sunday, I was going to go to church and dedicate my life to serving the Lord. I had been thinking about it but seeing my family and spending time with my grandmother was the final push I needed. Yep, I was done with the streets. Unfortunately, I never got a chance to head to church that Sunday or see my family again with my natural eyes. In less than twenty-four hours I would be blind with doctors saying there will be no recovery of my eyesight. I was to now navigate life as a blind man and see the side of God most with eyesight never see or experience. My life would never be the same.

Chapter 4: The Accident
Psalms 139:7-10

Although my father was not actively involved in my life during most of my childhood, we had created a strong bond as I got older. By the time I was in high school, we had become close as father and son and some would even say best friends. I enjoyed hunting and fishing with him as much as time allowed us to enjoy these sports. I was still primarily living with my grandparents throughout high school but would come up to spend weekends with my father in Pine Bluff. I liked staying with him because it gave me the freedom to do what I wanted to do without being under the watchful eyes of my grandparents. I could party, hang out and run the streets. As I had said before, even though my dad was a former police officer I made sure not to raise any suspicion with him as to my questionable activities. We had grown closer and I didn't want to mess that up or make him not trust me in his home. I made sure to keep my street drama away from him.

When I graduated from high school I moved in with my father, enrolled in college and found a job at a grocery store all while trying to build up my weed business. It was all quite a balancing act which I did very well. My father ended up accepting a job contract which required him to work overseas. It meant that I and my younger brother were living at his home and had the house to ourselves which was fine by me. My brother was my father's son by another woman but nonetheless we were growing quite close with one another. I didn't get him involved in my street hustle because I wanted to see him make something good of himself. By this time, I was growing tired of the streets myself and was ready to give it all up.

Although by this time I had a close bond with my father, I still had some disappointment with him and my mother for not making a strong enough effort in raising me. I felt that they left me and prioritized their own lives over being a parent to the child they created and brought into the world. This allowed for seeds of bitterness to grow within me. I never let them know how I felt because by that point in my life, I was officially of adult age and they could not make up for the years they lost during my childhood. I guess in a way my father felt that he was making up for those lost years by letting me stay and live with him. I appreciated him for it, but you can't take back painful memories of your childhood. They are imbedded within you forever. As close as my relationship with my father was evolving, the one with my mother was ever so turbulent. My mother and I stayed arguing and disputing about something. There was little to no peace between us. I wish I had a close relationship with my mother, but there was none.

When my father returned from his overseas work assignment, we picked up where we had left off. Dad and I both enjoyed gin and we'd drink, enjoy watching sports and hanging out together. One Saturday, he decided he wanted to go visit his parents over in Dumas, Arkansas which is almost a forty-five-minute drive. I enjoyed seeing and spending time with my other set of grandparents. Although I wasn't as close to them as I was with my maternal grandparents who'd raised me, being in their presence made me smile.

My grandmother was just as spiritual and religious as my other grandmother. She'd often admonish me about serving Jesus and staying on a righteous path. That Saturday during our visit with them, I remember my grandmother telling me that "God is good and Jesus is the only way". She would make sure you heard one of her mini-sermonettes before you left her house about the goodness of God. I didn't mind to hear her talk about the goodness of the Lord either. The irony was that just a day before my other grandmother had poured out her spiritual wisdom on me as well. Was God trying really hard to get my attention?

We spent a couple of hours with my grandparents but had to head back over to Pine Bluff to get ready for a party that evening. The son of my father's friend was turning three or four years old and wanted to celebrate it with a birthday party. It was also going to be a football watching party for us adults because there was a big game between the University of Arkansas Razorbacks and Auburn University's Tigers. College football is huge in the south and being that Arkansas did not have an NFL team, the Razorbacks had the devotion of thousands of fans within the state. I was looking forward to the game and hanging out with others. Although it was officially a children's birthday party, us adults were ready to enjoy some barbeque, beer and fun.

Dad and I got back from Dumas in time to pack the car up with some lawn chairs and a cooler full of drinks. By the time we ended up at the party the game was just about to start because it was a late afternoon, early evening start time. I knew some of the folks at the party but it was mainly friends of my father. Auburn was leading after the first quarter but couldn't keep up with the tenacious Arkansas offense for the rest of the game. Auburn didn't score another point after the first quarter and the Razorbacks won the game 38-14. Everybody was having a good time and things started to wind down around nine or ten.

Just as my father and I started packing the car up with our chairs and cooler one of his friends drove up. They engaged in a friendly taunting of one another about whose car was the fastest. Although we had come to the party in my father's truck, he also owned a 2002 supercharge Jaguar V8 and his friend was driving a 2011 Lexus who figured that since his car was the newest, he could win in a drag race and challenged my father to one. I had been a passenger in a few drag races with my dad and knew that his challenger may have bit off more than he could chew because that Jaguar was superfast. They agreed to meet back at the house we were about to leave and head over to a racing spot from there.

By the time we got back to the house my father was geeked and knew he could win the race. We had been talking about it during the ride home. We brought everything back into the house we had brought to the cookout and got ready for the race. Although I had been in a few races with him, something was telling me not to go and just sit this one out. I was sitting in the living room with my younger brother who had said he wanted to hang out with us because he wanted to get something to eat. He did not come to the party so I knew he was hungry. I thought we were going to leave right away but my father fiddled around in the back in his bedroom for about a half hour before we headed out of the door. By the time my father emerged from his bedroom I was still having some doubts about going but when he asked me if I was still going to come with him, I said "yes" without any hesitation. I told my brother to stay home and we'd bring him something back to eat. That right there perhaps saved his life.

My father's challenger called my father and changed plans to where we were to meet up. Rather than head back to the house where the party had been, he told us to meet him on this street which was a nice stretch for drag racing. I had been drinking but wasn't drunk. I never saw my father consume any alcohol during the party. By the time we got to the racing spot the other guy was already there waiting on us. They decided to race from one street light to the next. The street was a straight path and had two lanes but shifted to one lane that veered off onto the interstate. They lined their cars up at the light and as soon as the light turned green, they shot their cars forward like bullets leaving the chamber of a gun.

I remember looking at the speedometer of my father's car which read 155 mph. I was holding my cell phone in my hand but dropped it, maybe it was due to the high speed we were going. I unbuckled my seat belt to pick it up and tried to snap it back in place and looked over to my father. Would you believe that he had fallen asleep! We were still going well over 100 mph and the man was asleep. I yelled "Dad" real loud and hit him in the chest because I saw that we were about to hit a barrier. I grabbed the wheel and tried my best to steer the car to save us.

By this time my father had woke up and grabbed the steering wheel but it was too late. The car then flipped over several times but ended back on all four tires. We were still about to hit the barrel barriers and I braced for impact by grabbing the door. I know we hit those barriers while still going around 115 mph. I was thrown through the windshield head first and landed in a small ravine of water. I don't remember how long I was down in that water or how I managed to get up and walk out. I couldn't see anything but shadows and things were getting darker as I took each step. I was told that I was walking on the interstate with cars passing me by and I was heading into traffic when I was pulled back by a hand that grabbed my shoulder. It was my father's friend who had given the party that night.

I was walked back to his van and put in for the ride to the hospital. By this time my eyesight was just about gone and I could make out voices but not faces. I remember my dad's friend telling me to stay awake and not to die on him. I was in and out of consciousness, confused and in a lot of pain. My dad's friend dropped me off at the hospital and left. I was all alone. The hospital wasn't equipped to handle the injuries I had sustained and they did the best they could to get me stabilized in order to transfer me to a more equipped hospital. I was told that my head was split open to the point where you could see the brain matter and my eyes were popped out of their sockets, barely attached. I had cuts and bruises all over my body.

Apparently, my father was also in the van I was brought to the hospital in but refused to come in for treatment for his injuries. After about an hour, they transported me by ambulance to a larger hospital to begin surgery. By the time I got to the hospital several members of my mother's family including her were at the hospital. Them being there helped give me a little bit of peace. My grandfather said that all I kept telling them was that I wasn't driving and it wasn't my fault. I guess somehow, I felt they would blame it on me because they had known that I was out in the streets doing some wild things.

My mother was hurt, angry and afraid. I could hear it in her voice when she did approach me. Later I learned that when my father showed up at the hospital, she'd let him have it. She wanted to kill him for what he did. My mother denied him any visitation rights to see me at the hospital. To be honest, I am glad she did. Here I was a young man, blind and bruised by the actions of his father who didn't raise him as a child. I was young and reckless, but my father should have known better. It was later revealed to me that he had taken a sleeping pill just before the race which is why he fell asleep while driving. I know that the sleeping pills you get at the VA hospital are powerful so if he took one of those, I see why he was knocked out. That in and of itself lets you know that he was only thinking about himself to even race under those conditions. If I had known that, I know I would have stayed at the house.

When the doctor told me that I was blind and there was no possibility of recovery of my eyesight I did not want to believe it. I was confused, hurt and angry. Why me? Just the day before the accident I had told God that I was going to give my life over to Him. My plan was to go to church the next day, walk up to the altar and surrender my life over to the Lord. But now, here I was laid up in a hospital with no eyesight. I was a young man, barely in my twenties. The thought of not ever seeing the face of my daughter and family members was too much for me to take. This was unfair. Yes, I had done my dirt but none worse than the rest of the fools running the streets. This had to be a cruel joke, or a nightmare. I had my whole life ahead of me and now I was disabled. There was a lot that I had to process and accept, but I wasn't quite ready. I was angry at my father. I thought that if he had been a more responsible parent, he would have not ever let me drag race with him. But then again, I was an adult and got into that car under my own free will.

Laying up in a hospital bed will have you think about a lot of things. No matter how many times my mother and family members visited me, they still had to go home which meant that I was left alone to think. I was going over my life and thinking about the mistakes I made. I was thinking about how if I had listened to my spirit as I had so many times before I would have not gone on that ride with my father. Why did I ignore the warning? Was it my ego? Or was it the need to feel accepted by my father? There were so many questions. After periods of questioning things, I stopped asking and felt justified to be angry. Besides, who could blame me for being pissed off at the everyone?

Chapter 5: Hospital Stay

When I was transported to the hospital that was equipped to work on my injuries, I was rushed into a surgery that lasted seven hours. The surgeons had to remove my eyes in order to remove the pieces of glass that were in my sockets. There was a lot of glass they had to clean out. Although they did the best they could, I was still told that my blindness was permanent. It was the second or third day of my stay in the hospital when the physician came into my room to deliver that dreadful news. I remember my mother and one of my aunts being there with me when he said it. I recall my aunt going into prayer and saying that although the doctors are saying one thing, God will have the final say so and is still into performing miracles and healings. She has no idea how important that prayer was to me because it was finally sinking in that I needed a miracle for my eyesight to return.

I was angry, hurt and disappointed. My life was turned around in an instant. That car ride couldn't have been more than sixty-seconds, but the injuries would follow me for the rest of my life. My doctors all kept telling me to prepare to live my life as a blind man due to the extent of the injuries. I didn't want to hear any of that kind of talk. Up until that point I was an independent, strong and active young man. I couldn't imagine living the rest of my life dependent on other people. That thought left me angry and depressed. I'd do my best to put up a brave face when my family would come around and visit. But as soon as they left, my true feelings would take over. I did a lot of crying in that hospital bed.

On the second night of my stay I went into prayer asking God why did this happen to me. What happened next is not what I'd expected. I went into prayer going through what had become my regular mantra of complaints and questions to God – *Why did you let this happen to me? Why did you forsake me? Where were you God?* I was hurt and angry and didn't mind letting Him know it. Laying there in darkness in a hospital bed was not something I had planned on. It was unfair and cruel.

I let God have it until He finally had enough of my fussing, tears and anger. In the midst of one of my rants and melt downs, God spoke to me about the anger I was holding onto from childhood against my mother. God let me know that it was no accident that she didn't raise me nor was it a mistake. He said that He was in control the whole time and needed me to be raised by my grandparents. It was my grandparents who laid the spiritual foundation I needed for the call on my life. He knew I was special and had a special assignment on this earth. My grandparents protected me much better than my parents could have growing up. As if that was not enough, the Lord then showed me that so many people walk around with unforgiveness in their hearts and that is what leads them down a dark path of hopelessness. Some will die with that unforgiveness. I could have died the night of the accident with that same toxic unforgiveness imbedded in me. I know without a doubt I would have ended up, as the scriptures say, in an eternity of hell.

As if this were not enough, God then replayed to me the accident. Although I was a blind man, I could see in all clearly in my mind's eye. Every detail of the accident from first getting into the car and then flying through the windshield was revealed. It had to be God to show me this because up until that night I couldn't remember much about the accident. But laying there in the hospital bed, praying, crying and seeking it all came back to me. I saw my father, I recall the conversation, I felt the fear, and realized the impact of the crash on my body. It was a lot for me to take in, but I needed for God to do this. I needed to know that I still had a purpose and that nothing happens coincidently. I ultimately asked God to forgive me for my anger towards my parents and Him. I repented and made the choice to move ahead with my life. I had the greatest intentions, but what was to come was not going to be easy.

Chapter 6: Accepting My New Life as a Blind Man

I was released from the hospital after the third day of my stay. The doctors had done all they could and sent me home. By the time of my discharge, I had peace with my parents and myself. I was no longer bitter and angry towards my mother or father. I also had to forgive myself because up until that point I had been blaming myself for the accident. I had to also release my father from his responsibility in the accident and forgive him. Although he did not go to jail for what he did, I kept him imprisoned in my mind because of my anger. I had to let that anger towards him go. By the time my grandfather and mother came to the hospital to take me home, I felt as if a heavy burden had been lifted. I was ready to live and make the best of my life.

The people at the hospital were pretty nice to me for the most part but I wasn't given anything as an aid to help me as a blind man. I left the hospital with no cane to try and feel my way around a room. My grandparents moved me into their new home which was not the home I had lived in with them. The layout was a bit different so it took me a minute to figure out how to get around the rooms. A few times I'd bump into things and would get angry. My balance was the hardest thing to deal with because I'd often lose my balance and would fall. You'd be surprised to learn how important eyesight is in keeping you balanced on your feet. My grandparents did the best they could to help me get adjusted to the home. I appreciated the love and kindness they showed towards me.

Now that I was no longer the street hustler out there on the party scenes, my friends were far and few between. I didn't have many visitors and the ones that would come by were typically relatives. My grandmother kept me company with her inspiring and truthful conversations. I remember her telling me that the night of the accident, she was called and told that I was now blind and she hung the phone up on the person. She did not want to hear that her baby boy could no longer see. I know she went into deep prayer that night because that is what my grandma would always do in times of a crisis.

There were many moments of weeping I did while staying with my grandparents. When no one was home, and I was left to my own thoughts I would sink into a deep depression.

After a while though, I could no longer pretend to be ok to the world. Depression became my main state of existence. I'd cry and stayed locked up in my bedroom. I didn't want to be around anybody and was tired. I was literally now fighting for my life because I did not want to live. Although I was still a young man, I felt old and useless inside. My eyesight was an important part of what made me who I was, or so I thought. My ability to make money had depended on my eyesight. Now that it was gone, I felt useless. I convinced myself that I could not be a provider for my daughter and that no woman would ever want to deal with a blind man. The more I thought on these things the deeper I fell into depression. I had lost the will to live and didn't think my purpose on the earth was needed anymore.

The thing about depression is that it has a strong way of convincing you that hopelessness is your only fate. It will tell you that you are better off dead than alive. I had been fighting a lot of suicidal thoughts and wanted to die. I'd be sitting in the middle of the floor rocking back and forth in silence. If someone came into the room and touched me, I'd jump in fear. One day, while my grandparents were out running errands, I listened to the voices in my head to just go on and kill myself. Before I realized it, I headed into the kitchen and grabbed a long knife with the intent of stabbing myself and bleeding out. I fumbled through the drawer until I got ahold of the knife and pressed it in my stomach. It was if a hand had grabbed mine and wouldn't let me push the knife further in. I pulled my hand back and tried it a second time. The same thing happened, the knife wouldn't go any further. That's when I realized that it was not meant for me to die that day and I put the knife down, fell on the floor and cried for about an hour before making my way back into my bed to cry some more. Not even death would grant me what I wanted that day.

The next day my 3-year-old daughter came into the room, as she would always do. I turned my back away from her and would face the wall. I felt helpless that I couldn't do the things I wanted to do with her as her father now that I was blind. Like an angel sent from heaven, that day she touched me on my shoulder and said "Daddy, you're going to see again". I then turned over to face her, and asked her what did you say. She repeated it, "Daddy you're going to see again". That was the most powerful thing anybody had said to me since the accident. I grabbed her and held her tight. From that day forward, I had a little hope and was able to face her and play with her when she came around. The scripture says in Psalms 8:2, "Out of the mouth of babes and sucklings hast thou ordained strength." That day, my baby girl gave me the strength to live, she gave me purpose again.

From that day forward, I knew that my life would not be easy. Regardless, I had determination and purpose. For the first time since the accident I was beginning to learn how to live again. I knew that I was not the only person in the world who had lost their eyesight and there had been many blind people who went on to do some great things. I knew that in the darkness I was now living in, it was my call to bring people into the light. I was to bring hope to the hopeless and comfort to the comfortless. It was time for Briston Bailey to be the man he had always been called to be. It was time for me to live out my purpose.

Chapter 7: Answering the Call

Prior to my accident I had made up my mind to live for Christ. I'm not going to lie and say that it was an easy and smooth decision. As you already know, there were a lot of temptations I had to separate myself from in order to be really committed. Perhaps if I did not lose my eyesight I may not have been as committed to serving the Lord, or perhaps it would not have made a difference. Let me tell you though that giving your life to Christ versus accepting the call on your life to be committed to the work of the ministry are miles apart.

There is a very high level of accountability when you walk in the office of ministry. You are literary responsible for countless souls who are watching your walk and sitting under your teachings. There are many ministers who say one thing in the pulpit but live an entirely different life behind closed door. I didn't want to be one of those ministers. I've never been the type of man to live a hypocritical life and I wasn't about to start it once I became a minister.

Although I was saved, it was still a struggle for me to accept my call but I finally did in

November 2012, just before I became a student at the school of the blind. I will never forget that day. I stood in front of the church and committed myself to the service of Christ, it was at a midweek Wednesday service. Just prior to that day I remember being in my bedroom struggling with answering the call. I had a lot of questions, fears and apprehensions. I didn't know how the people would accept a blind man preaching in the pulpit. My confidence was at an all-time low and I was still fighting occasional bouts of depression. In spite of all of that, I began to study and read God's word through my braille bible. Soon, I realized that I was cut from a different cloth and of a different breed. I began to understand and accept that I was called to be a prophet of God.

From the age of sixteen to twenty-two, my life was a wrestling match with God. The more God pressed upon me that I was called to deliver His word the more I pushed away. There were a lot of things my flesh still enjoyed such as drinking, partying, getting high, hustling, multiple women, cussing, etc. I knew that I had to give up those things once the call on my life was accepted. I didn't want to give any of it up. I was blind, but still liked to have fun if the opportunity presented itself.

One day though, God showed me in a vision the replay of my car accident but this time it was from the vantage point of the spiritual messages and meanings of it. That's when I finally saw my higher purpose on this earth and that my life was spared for a divine reason. The weight of the call on my life fell heavy on me because I had no idea how I'd accomplish any of it. I broke down in tears and let God know that I couldn't do any of it by himself. I asked God to be by my side to help me and show me the way to go on a righteous path. Soon after, I publicly accepted my call and it was not too far along that I finally understood that you pay a heavy price for that call and spiritual gift. In my case it cost me my eyesight.

I will never forget the first sermon I had preached which I gave two and a half months after accepting my call. It was given on Superbowl Sunday in 2013. It was delivered in the church my grandparents were members of which I had joined. Several members of my family were in attendance and despite it being a being Superbowl Sunday and the weather not being the best (very cold), the church still had a good number of people in attendance. My sermon was called "Kill All the Flesh till The Flesh Kills You" (I Samuel 15). It was centered on when God told Saul to kill all of the Amalekites, but he didn't obey and just killed what he thought was good and ended up dying himself. It was a powerful lesson on why it's important to obey the instructions of God in your life and not compromise because it could cost you everything.

I had become a member of the church and grew close with the pastor. I am forever grateful to him because he gave me my first opportunity to preach in public. He was my mentor as well as my pastor. My pastor would help me navigate through biblical questions I had. I enjoyed being at the church but outgrew it after about four months. I was a fulltime student at the school of the blind which was forty-five minutes away from the church. Being that I was no longer able to drive, I had to depend on others to bring me to church. After a while, transportation became too much of a burden and I had to make a choice.

Prior to that though something happened that lined up with my destiny. One Sunday I was delivering a sermon and in attendance was another pastor who was sitting in the back. He didn't stay until the end of the sermon and left before the service was done. Although I knew him, I didn't connect with this pastor until four months later and what he told me shook my soul. He said that as he listened to me preach, the Lord spoke to him and told him that I was too raw for the church I was in and that my time was up for me to remain. Ultimately, I ended up in his church and he became my pastor.

Joining that church has changed my life. I'm still a member of the church as at the time of the writing of this book. My pastor has opened up a spiritual world to me that has helped me to sharpen my prophetic gift. I've spent many hours with him which has given me better confidence as a minister. Sometimes you don't realize what you need until it happens. I was content in my old church but wasn't growing at the pace I needed to be. At that time, I didn't see it, but my current pastor did. When I first started attending, my pastor would let me preach here and there.

Eventually I began to grow into my gift with more confidence and was given more opportunities to preach. I even had requests to come and preach at other churches. I'm beginning to see the truth in the scripture found in Proverbs 18:16 which says, "A man's gift maketh room for him, and bringeth him before great men." The more I preach the more the prophetic in me flows out.

Eventually my pastor told me that it was time to become ordained in ministry. I had already been licensed through my former pastor but this was the next big step. I will never forget my ordination service. It was me and another minister who had to pass an oral biblical exam in front of the entire church. The other minister and I were very nervous but we passed. I was grateful, excited and humbled. The long journey to finally walk in my office as a prophet was officially on paper through my ordination papers. God was true to His word and showed me the greatest love and patience I had ever experienced.

Chapter 8: The Future Looks Brighter Than Ever

One thing I can tell you for sure and that is God is faithful and will NEVER forsake you no matter how dark life appears. In less than ten years I went from a man who wanted to end his life to one who is happy and sees a bright future ahead of him. My life has not always been easy, but it has taught me that through faith and perseverance, you can achieve anything.

I also now have a beautiful wife in my life. Just prior to me getting engaged my mind became centered on developing a relationship with a God-fearing woman. I believe that we are on the planet to honor God and also cultivate relationships with others. Not everyone will get or desire to be married, but we all have to interact with other people in some capacity. In order for me to build a solid relationship with a woman, I had to become whole within myself first. Through time spent with God's word, mentoring from my pastor and learning to adjust to life as a blind man I had released a lot of the anger and hurt that were holding me back. I was back in love with my life and wanted to share it with someone else as my wife.

I dated a few women but after a short period I knew it would not have worked because they couldn't see themselves in a long-term relationship with a man with a disability. Although I was very independent and learned how to do a lot of things on my own, I knew that in the back of these women's minds they felt that I would be more of a burden on them. I didn't want a wife who felt as if I was a burden so we ended those relationships.

One day while attending a single's seminar at our church a young lady was brought to my attention by my pastor. He and I were sitting in his truck when all of a sudden he said out loud, "I think I see the next Mrs. Bradley". He described her to me and I liked what I heard but didn't approach her at all during the seminar. She was a member of our church and a faithful believer in Jesus Christ. About three weeks after the seminar, God spoke to me to approach her and officially meet her. I believe if God hadn't intervened, I would have never approached her. I was never the shy type of guy but with my disability and having no good luck with the women I had been dating, I was apprehensive in stepping to her.

I had been playing the drums at church and decided that it was the day to speak to her. After service, I got up from the drum set and asked someone nearby where she was at so that I could approach her. It so happened that she was walking towards my direction so I called out her name to get her attention. I formally introduced myself to her, engaged in some small talk and asked for her number. I asked her if she was afraid that I was blind and she let me know that she had a grandmother who was visually impaired and it didn't bother her. Great, this was a perfect start!

We had a few phone conversations and would see one another at church. I invited her out on what would be our first date and let her pick the restaurant. From there we'd go on other dates including the movies (yes, blind people can enjoy the movies too), restaurants, fishing and church activities. I was feeling her and she was feeling me. Our relationship had grown close to the point where one day she broke down and told me that she was hurt in the past and wanted to be spiritual and grow more in God. Soon after, during some prayer time, God spoke to me that I was sent into her life to help her with spiritual growth. I know also that she's in my life to help me to see things about myself I had not seen before. She's showed me faithfulness, unconditional love and what it takes to build a marriage.

We dated for about a year when I knew for sure this woman was to be my wife. On the day of my ordination, after passing my oral exam before the entire church I called her up to the front. I thanked her for her support, got on one knee, presented her with a ring that I picked out with her father and asked if she'd marry me. She was surprised and happy. We got married a year later in 2017. This beautiful woman, Phoebe, who became my wife has since given me my second child. We're the proud parents of a beautiful baby girl. Now, we've had our moments of disagreements and growth but I know that there's a purpose for our marriage.

In spite of all that I've gone through, I know that the ministry is what I will be serving for the remainder of my life. I am so grateful to God for His patience and love shown to me. I don't know how my life would have ended up if I hadn't lost my sight. Perhaps I would have become faithful in the church for a short while and then fall back to the ways of street ways, who knows. All I know is that right now my future is looking bright and I have a clear vision. I have risen from that dark place of violence, disobedience and hell.

I enjoy the ministry but I don't see myself as a pastor for some years. Walking in the office of a prophet is where I am supposed to be for right now. I know that my call will help to sanitize the gift of the prophetic. I am an endstime prophet here to deliver a word of truth to God's people. The word I deliver is raw and the dreams and visions I receive are anointed. In spite of my gift, it's important for me to remain humble and grateful for each day. I do not want to become one who is so puffed up in my office that I can no longer relate to the people I'm ministering to and think that I'm above them. That is sacrilegious.

The gift of a prophet on my life has been confirmed through signs and wonders. One Sunday, my pastor let me hold a service at the church and a lady came in and I ministered to her. In a vision, I saw that this woman had some children and that she had one who was heading into some danger. I told her that the child was in their early twenties and the woman confirmed that her daughter was twenty-one and was living a very wild life. I told the woman if the young lady didn't turn her life around, she'd meet an early death. It shook the woman but she was grateful for the warning. This is one of many instances of God using my gift to help and empower people. Some so-called prophets may be afraid to deliver such a harsh word to the people, but that isn't me.

I've been blessed to be touched and inspired by some men of God who have gone through all kinds of ups and downs in their ministry. Here are just a few that I admire and see as mentors:

1) Benny Hinn – he has an awesome worship atmosphere, he operates in miracles in his gift of healing.

2) Rod Parsley – his rawness and heartfelt outreach for the people of God changes lives.

3) Prophet Brian Carn – he is powerful with how he flows in worship and let's God use him through the anointing on his life. The anointing you respect is the anointing you attract. He has a strong deliverance ministry.

4) My Pastor of Greater Works Christian Church (Little Rock), Pastor Micheal E. Clayton – he operates in the five-fold ministry with the apostolic ways very heavy on his life. He operates in miracles, healings and deliverance. He's my mentor who has taken me under his wings when others

passed over me. He's groomed me by way of the Holy Ghost into the prophetic during this time and in my lifetime. He's showed me unconditional acceptance and love.

The vision I have for my ministry and movement is to open people's eyes through God's word and the gift He's placed on my life. I envision that my call will also bring unity, help to erase racism and division which this nation has suffered from for far too long, bring young people back to God and let them know that there is hope for their future. I pray that God will continue to use me to show people that no matter how bad life may be to them, there is always hope. I've overcome much and am here to let the people know that there is always hope and a future.

Lastly, I want to share a message to any young man that will read this book. I want you to know that being different will actually be the best thing that ever happens to you. It pays to be on God's side. The world has a system, (John 17), that is set up for us to be damned to hell because the world cannot teach us the worldly perspective to make it to heaven. I pray that you take the time to find a church that is truly operating in the power of God and has His presence operating all of the time. Put the same energy into finding a church home as you did to find the biggest party and newest club. There's nothing in this world worth losing your life for, only God. I've seen the worst in this world – have had friends forsake me, people take from me and others who've lie. I've lost my eyesight because of some poor decisions. This is what the world does, it's a dog eat dog world.

I am begging you to listen. Even though you will go through some things during your Christian walk, God always makes it better. The blessings will triumph anything you go through. Leave the streets alone because there's nothing but death and destruction in them. If you ever need anyone to call on first let me recommend Jesus, then a pastor that has God's heart. Also, be careful of the communication you keep. Some of you reading this book are thinking of switching your friends, and I admonish you to don't hesitate. God is reaching for you. God is crying for you to come to Him. There is nothing better than giving your life to Christ, that's the only thing that saved my life and I am forever grateful for it. If you ever think you can't be loved, God loves you and I most definitely love you too. May God bless you all!

Made in United States
Orlando, FL
18 March 2025